DEEP-SENSORY

If you are highly sensitive

Advisor

Gudrun Leyendecker

Biographical information from the German National Library: The German National Library lists this publication in the German National Bibliography; detailed biographical data is available on the Internet at http://dnb.dnb.de.

Translation: Deepl/ Birte Micheels

© 2024 Gudrun Leyendecker

Production and publisher: BoD - Books on Demand, Norderstedt

ISBN: 9 783 759 758 835

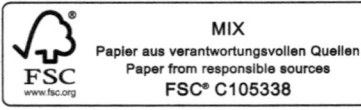

The book DEEP-SENSORY with the subtitle: "If you are highly sensitive",

shows questions and answers for people who have problems with their sensitivity.

It is estimated that between 15 and 30% of people belong to the group of highly sensitive people due to their sensitive perception.

Among them are people who have to find their own way to find their place in today's struggle for existence. Many of them are not aware that this subtle disposition can also be a gift.

Gudrun Leyendecker has been an author since 1995. She was born in Bonn in 1948.

See Wikipedia.

She has published around 98 books, including non-fiction, crime novels, romance novels and satire. Leyendecker also writes as a ghostwriter for well-known directors. She is a member of writers' associations and an Italian cultural association. She also gained experience for her work during her decades as a life counselor.

DEEP-SENSORY

If you are highly sensitive

Advisor

Gudrun Leyendecker

For RIKE

In deep solidarity

Topics and keywords in this book:

- High sensitivity is neither an illness nor a mental disorder
- I wish I was an elephant
- Why I am writing this book
- my learned experiences
- Deep-sensory
- Sensitivity and resilience in everyday life
- Tips for the evening
- the sleep
- Tips for the morning
- leisure time
- a few suggestions to get creative
- A few advantages and disadvantages of high sensitivity
- What is positive stress?
- Example for ...
- A great advantage that a highly sensitive person has ...
- all our senses have...

- Different types where high sensitivity is a particular issue
- the order fanatic
- the anxious type
- the word fear... tightness
- the you-man
- the fear biter
- the restless, the hectic
- the hermit
- the panic attacks
- feel powerless
- we practise pondering
- We should only worry about things ...
- The feeling
- The dreams
- Quick help
- get creative
- Goethe, poem about feelings
- Self-love and love
- Love yourself with flaws and weaknesses

- The highly sensitive person in the partnership
- Moods
- all feelings are allowed
- Anger
- the laughter
- Joy

If you have found something that interests you and possibly affects you in some way, it makes sense to read on.

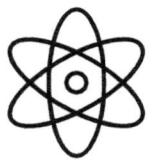

High sensitivity is neither an illness nor a mental disorder. A highly sensitive person is characterized by an extremely intense perception of all sensory

stimuli. Some or all of their senses are very sensitive and these people process all perceptions very thoroughly. Because of this ability, I also classify this type of person as deeply sensitive. Further reasons and explanations can be found on the following pages.

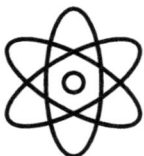

Many people I have met over the many decades of my life and still meet today suffer from their high sensitivity. They feel like a marginalized group, sometimes excluded from the group of people who are more or less carefree, courageous and largely fearless in their pursuit of various goals.

Because highly sensitive people process everything very thoroughly, they often need more time and, above all, more energy to do so.

The basic requirement for highly sensitive people is to ensure that their nervous strain does not get out of hand.

Due to the greater effort that highly sensitive people need to process, they are generally more quickly exhausted and less resilient.

Because of the sensitivity of his perceptions, he usually feels rather "annoyed", irritated and burdened, and his feelings do not deceive him. The limit of his resilience lies far below the resilience of those people who are not highly sensitive and are equipped with a "thick nervous system" or, as they say in the vernacular, a "thick skin".

In order not to be disadvantaged as a highly sensitive person, it is important to recognize yourself, accept yourself and learn to live positively with your high sensitivity.

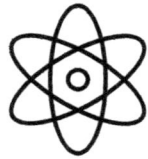

As a child, I heard my father say the saying that I still remember today:

I wish I was an elephant,

then I would cheer loudly:

It wouldn't be because of the ivory

No, because of the thick skin.

I think this saying comes from a highly sensitive person who wanted to have a good nervous system and who did not feel comfortable among less sensitive people. I also gather from these words that this poet felt disadvantaged and could not really use his high sensitivity in a positive way. He envied the less sensitive people and obviously suffered from the disadvantages that a highly sensitive person can have. But this is exactly where every highly sensitive person can start. They have the opportunity to live more intensively and better in a positive way and can discover the creative potential that they can draw from their soul.

The deeply processed impressions contain a great potential for creative ideas. Everything a person has experienced finds an echo in their soul.

Many people claim that they are not creative, but everyone can awaken something in themselves that allows creativity to flow (more on this later in this book).

Believers are convinced that they were created by (a) God in his image. It is therefore also understandable that there is creative power in every human being, even if it is sometimes (still) hidden.

And with all this knowledge about highly sensitive people and being able to draw on my creative potential, I am quite sure that being a highly sensitive person is good for me. I don't want to have the proverbial "thick skin", no "elephant skin" as my skin. I like my sensitive skin.

Rainer Maria Rilke

expresses his feelings, his high
sensitivity in a poem:

*If only it would be, just once,
completely quiet.*

*If the random and, the
approximate*

*Went mute, and the neighbors'
laughter,*

If the noise that my senses
make,

Would not so stubbornly keep
me from waking,

-

Then I could, in a thousandfold

Thought, think you right to the
edge of you

and have you (just a smile
long),

to give to all life as a gift

like a thank-you.

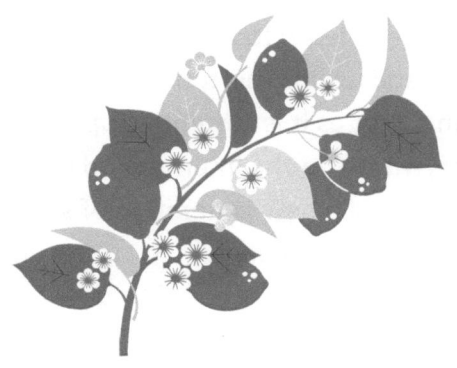

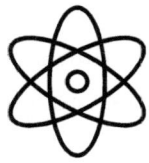

Take a break! Look at a flower or a leaf
(if it is possible, in nature), see how
creative nature is!

Why am I writing this book?

The topic of high sensitivity is important. Especially in these fast-moving times, we have to learn to reflect on ourselves again and again. This topic seems to be brand new, as it is currently appearing everywhere on the internet and in the media, as if a new generation of special people has been born.

Highly sensitive people have been around for ages, but their abilities have rarely been noticed, often even less appreciated and sometimes even tabooed. Especially in this day and age of widespread communication through the media, this taboo should be broken. It is important that the different groups of people understand each other and get to know each other.

It is particularly important that people who belong to the group of highly sensitive people connect with each other in order to exchange ideas and share similarities. But it is just as important that the group of less sensitive people not only shows understanding for the highly sensitive people, but also enables them to act in positions where they can give their best. The less sensitive people must learn to be more considerate, more attentive, more mindful, especially when living together with the highly sensitive people.

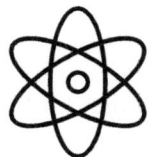

As I grew up in an environment of highly sensitive people and was often surrounded by them later in life, I, 76 years old, report al lot of life experiences.

Sensitivity is not a disease, but a special disposition that you should recognize and accept in yourself in order to learn how to deal with it correctly.

My own story is a life with high sensitivity.

Some readers may find themselves in this report and receive suggestions for living their own life of high sensitivity.

I was born in 1948, in the post-war period, as the fourth child in a family of artists.

My mother was not only a pianist and highly gifted musician, she also had a talent for drawing and writing poetry. Because of her own sensitivity, she suffered from migraines for many decades of her life, had stomach ulcers and gallstones. All these manifestations of the body indicate that the artist was too stressed by everyday and other problems.

My father, an art historian and doctor of philosophy, also played the piano, painted, wrote poetry and wrote art history travel guides. He suffered from high blood pressure and cardiac arrhythmia for many years, which later led to him being fitted with a pacemaker. This is also a sign that he was constantly exposed to too many stressful moments.

Even though the word "highly sensitive" wasn't used back then, I am convinced that both my parents should be counted as highly sensitive people.

My mother always worried a lot about us, which she shared with us. My eldest sister's illness, who suffered from various symptoms of a mental disorder on her way to adulthood, was a particularly hard blow. I was sensitized to the sensitive people around me and to people with symptoms of illness.

I remember the first moments of fear in my life: alone in a dark room, fear of various adults, vague feelings of anxiety.

Asthma in early childhood led to lung sensitivity, followed by whooping cough, two bouts of pneumonia and pleurisy as a child. An aversion to milk and butter made me avoid these products. I often developed nausea when driving, apparently a reaction of "the sense of balance".

I didn't go to kindergarten, but invented a lot of fantasy games, as my older siblings were already at school at the time and I was often left to my own devices, for example when my mother wasn't feeling well. I invented friends who didn't exist, fantasized and played with non-existent people.

As I was still quite a good student in elementary school, my fears were limited during this time, especially as I soon discovered that there were a few things I could do better than many others. These were drawing, painting, writing stories and the ability to empathize with others. This led me to acting in amateur theater groups at an early age. Wherever the opportunity arose, I played various roles. My sister and I often performed sketches, small or larger plays, which we presented to any audience.

From the 5th school year, my first year at grammar school, I put myself under pressure to perform. Various fears prevented me from expressing myself. Fear of failure was combined with a fundamental fear of making mistakes and the fear of embarrassing myself in front of my classmates.

At the same time, I had joined a circle of new classmates, almost all of whom belonged to an upper class. There were many girls in my class, some of whose parents were important personalities and, above all, very wealthy. These schoolgirls attached great importance to their appearance, their image and everything material.

However, I had already been presented with a particular ideology for idealistic values at home and had been shown that it was a goal worth striving for. This made me fit in very poorly with my classmates, especially the elite clique that had formed a special group.

It was all about parties, model dresses and other fashion.

There were only a few classmates who thought like me and very few who felt like me. I had a casual acquaintance with these classmates, and a deep and genuine friendship with only one of them, which still exists today.

My friend and I had ambivalent feelings about being excluded and ridiculed by the others. On the one hand, there was the desire to be included in the group of famous girls in the elite class; on the other hand, I was happy with my little talents, which allowed me to be different and earned me praise from others.

While my sister's illness continued to affect our family's life, my grades at school got noticeably worse.

In addition, I was very disappointed when I found out that life is not all fair. Everything pointed to the fact that grades are not always distributed fairly and not according to performance. Rumor had it that the influential parents of the VIP girls did everything, including illicit things, to get their daughters good grades. This experience depressed me.

During a brief, indifferent phase of depression in puberty, I visited a psychotherapist twice, who was still called a "neurologist" at the time. After a few sessions, I felt better again.

My desire for independence and a family in which I wanted to realize my dream of a harmonious life together led me to get married at the age of 20. I became the mother of two children at the age of 21 and 23.

But in the meantime, I had unconsciously adopted a way of behaving that bought me peace wherever I went: I usually aligned myself with other people and avoided arguments and fights. I kept the house of cards of my first partnership standing for over 23 years by being diplomatic and keeping a low profile. Only when it came to the children could I be the fighting lioness.

After stomach ulcers and a recommended therapy with a psychotherapist, I slowly came to the realization that things were going wrong in my life and that I needed a change.

After the divorce, it wasn't long before I got married again. But I still hadn't learned to pay enough attention to myself and my high sensitivity.

I worked too many hours as a life coach, sometimes even at night, and so I maneuvered myself into an extremely severe burnout at the age of 63.

A blood pressure that was far too high could not be treated satisfactorily in hospital, and I had panic attacks as a result.

After a year of good therapeutic counseling, I started to feel better and was able to look to the future with hope. After three years of good and regular treatment with a behavioral therapist and a visit to the cardiologist, I was able to stop taking the medication.

I was also able to learn to better recognize the interplay between my soul, psyche and body. In the years that followed, I also practiced how to instruct my own body to listen to its own instructions. First of all, I started with breathing exercises and relaxation exercises.

The effects on my body showed me how well it works with me when I instruct it.

Over the next few years, I learned to pay attention not only to my gut feeling, but to every indication my body gave me.

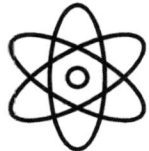

My learned experiences

If you listen to your body language, you will perceive the wake-up calls and warnings of your own body. Through various types of tension, it tells us that we need to relax. (Headaches, muscle tension, back pain, various aches and pains, anxiety, etc.)

To relax, you should choose the right activities or hobbies (breathing therapies, meditation, creative hobbies, sport, etc.). See specifically the following pages on hobbies etc.

It is not only interesting, but also good and strengthening to feel how well and quickly the body reacts and that you can "govern" it.

The feeling of having your body "under control" is a feeling of strength and boosts self-confidence.

As I now also consider my high sensitivity to be a gift, I feel that I have a duty to treat this gift with gratitude.

It gives rise to great creativity, which I want to protect.

To protect them, I have to seek stress relief, relaxation, after every stress.

To protect this gift, I take great care to feed my soul and psyche with soul food.

A walk in nature, a short activity with an animal or child, communication with a loved one, a short sporting exercise, meditation, a creative activity brings me back into harmony, into physical and mental balance.

Of course, life always brings new tasks, new problems and also strokes of fate that you can't avoid.

You have to know that you can always be brought back to a point where you have to start all over again, to reflect, to find yourself and to rebuild yourself positively.

Since life has a changing rhythm in everything (inhale and exhale, day and night, etc.), you are constantly faced with new challenges that you can face.

These challenges strengthen the soul, psyche and body and weave a net for immunization, so to speak.

A fundamental attitude to life is important here. Many people feel that they are being pursued by bad luck and are frustrated, assuming that life or people have something against them.

A healthy attitude is based on the learning effect. Every experience, whether positive or negative, can lead to a strengthening of self-confidence if it has been properly processed. Everything that we have successfully overcome and learned from is a basis of experience that can strengthen and protect us for the future.

We can reinforce this effect by praising ourselves. And not just for major successes, but for everything we achieve.

This is especially true for activities that we don't like doing, that we have aversions to. It is not always possible to avoid them, but we should be aware that everything we do is voluntary. Because if we don't want to do something, we can say "no".

We should not only praise ourselves after an activity that we don't like, but also relax. Over time, we also learn to trust our gut feeling and take precautions, preferably before our body tells us that we are doing something that is not good for us.

We become more and more mindful when we start to listen more to our feelings and intuition and especially to our body language.

This mindfulness should become as natural to us as daily hygiene (I have summarized the spiritual cleansing through washing rituals in another book with advice: Making You Feel Good).

Dealing with our high sensitivity requires caution and patience and some practice. The older we are, the more negative things we have accumulated, the longer the learning process can take and the more patient we have to be with ourselves.

Even at an advanced age, you are not too old, we should always be open to new insights that bring us improvement. Everyone should keep an open mind so that they ultimately have the opportunity to make life more enjoyable and successful for themselves.

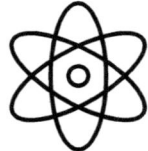

DEEP-SENSORY

The title of this book is the key word for dealing with high sensitivity.

We use the word "profound" when a person thinks deeply, ponders something, thinks profoundly, seeks meaning in a matter and moves their thoughts into the depths. "Sense" and "pondering" are a clear characteristic of mental, intellectual work.

However, we must not forget that the word "sense" also has something to do with the related word "sense" (senses), in the meaning of our sensory organs.

Most people are aware of their seven senses, which enable them to hear, see, taste, smell, touch, feel and keep their bodies in balance.

Becoming aware of this deep sensitivity in two senses is the task of highly sensitive people. It is important to recognize and accept your predisposition and find ways to enrich your life with this predisposition.

Every person is an individual.

And you also know that the development of these senses can vary greatly.

Highly sensitive people often have particularly intense "feeling" senses, which can be very sensitive, sometimes even delicate.

This group of people, the size of which is not entirely clear (it varies between approx. 15 and 30 %), includes both "deep thinkers" and "deep feelers".

There are now tests that can be used to determine high sensitivity.

As a rule, you realize this in the course of your life at the latest when your high sensitivity leads to problems or illnesses.

On the following pages you will find examples of people with high sensitivity and tips on how to deal with this predisposition and how to integrate it into your life.

Unfortunately, even in this day and age, there is still far too much taboo surrounding both the psyche and sensitivity. Even in this century, seeing a therapist for a mental disorder is unfortunately still not a matter of course.

On the following pages I would like to familiarize both highly sensitive people and those around them with the typical characteristics, add explanations and encourage further thoughts.

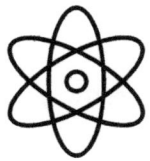

Sensitivity and resilience

Everyday life

Highly sensitive people have a stronger sensory perception, which is also reflected in the individual sensory organs.

A sensitive person may not only have a thinner nervous system, but may also be more strongly affected by the external stimuli that touch their sensory organs, and may also be under greater strain.

Sensitive people are often less able to tolerate noise and disturbing sounds, as well as various light influences and reflections. Smells can also be perceived as more disturbing, and touching the skin is perceived more intensely.

As all sensory organs have extremely sensitive "antennae", sensory overload during everyday life can lead to stress and disturbances. Sensitive people should protect themselves as much as possible from this overload. This is often not possible in everyday life, so sensitive people need extensive body and soul care at the end of the day to relieve their tense nerves and overstimulated sensory organs. Taking time for this is extremely important.

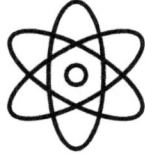

Tips for the evening:

I remember from my childhood the evening walk that many people took before going to bed. Nowadays, people sometimes go jogging; depending on the type of person, fast walking can also provide relief for stressed people. Gentle dance movements accompanied by relaxing music help to reduce tension.

A contemplative walk is also particularly useful for sensitive people, as it is not only good for the body, but also for the soul. Small paths into nature are ideal, as they can offer neutralizing images to the hectic daily routine.

Large meals in the late evening put a strain on the body and also prevent sensitive people's stomachs from settling down. A small, easily digestible snack in the early evening, on the other hand, has a positive effect.

After an evening washing ceremony (bath or shower) and relaxation rituals, it is beneficial to free yourself from the excitement and anger of the day. Depending on your taste, you can enjoy a good book, relaxing music or sparing use of media in a relaxing form.

It is recommended that you only go to bed when you are really tired. Highly sensitive people often have many circling thoughts that prevent them from falling asleep even though they are tired. It is often good to review the day in order to come to terms with what has happened. Rituals or prayers can be used to clear the mind of the remaining stressful thoughts.

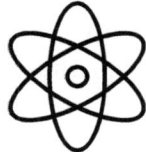

Sleep:

Any excitement before sleep should be avoided; instead, regular relaxation times are beneficial for "coming down" into a mental balance.

It's better to be completely tired first, or to "tire yourself out" instead of lying awake in bed brooding!

Don't find waking up at night annoying! There were times when people used to eat something at night or pursue their hobbies. You could read, write, paint, do crossword puzzles, etc.

Going for a walk indoors or on the balcony or in the garden in warm weather can also have a relaxing effect.

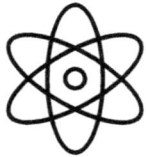

Tips for the morning:

Early morning gymnastics, a morning prayer, a long shower and a walk bring body and soul into a good balance.

Every person has their own individual resilience. For a highly sensitive person, the sensory overload of everyday life is often too great a stress factor.

What can be done? The ideal solution would be work that is individually tailored to the sensitive person, not too many hours a day and with plenty of breaks.

This is generally not feasible.

Many people are in a job that neither touches on their talents nor matches their dispositions.

In short, a highly sensitive person often works in a stressful environment (noises, uncomprehending colleagues, uncomprehending bosses), performs work that does not suit them

and is also under pressure to succeed.

Most people work for a living and therefore cannot easily give up their job.

Reducing working hours is often not feasible for this reason either.

Solution tips:

Relaxation breaks must be built in.

Alternatively, additional relaxation space must be created during leisure time.

Hobbies that are individually tailored to highly sensitive people must be given more space in their free time.

Art and creativity are valuable tools for relaxing and unwinding.

Ideally, you should switch to a suitable occupation, but as this is not possible in most cases, the suitable activity is shifted to your free time.

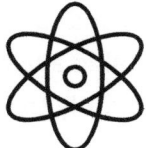

The leisure time

You don't have to be an artist to live out your creativity in your free time.

There are certainly many highly sensitive people among painters, sculptors and talented draughtsmen, but there is a huge spectrum of fields of activity in which you can live out your sensitivity creatively without being an artist.

Here are a few suggestions:

It starts in the kitchen, because there are no constraints when it comes to baking, cooking and inventing recipes. Preserving and making syrups and juices has also become very fashionable again. Baking dough can be used not only to make beautiful gifts, but also pretty accessories.

There are also no limits to creativity when it comes to the garden, balcony or houseplants. Whether it's a vegetable patch or growing flowers, your own tomato bush on the balcony or cacti in the living room and growing in a mini-greenhouse, here you can watch life develop and flourish under your care.

Handicrafts, starting with sewing, embroidery, crocheting and knitting, offer a great field of activity for relaxation. What was a matter of course for women in other centuries is now accessible to all genders and serves (in moderation) as a diversion and relaxation.

When crafting with any material, you can let your creativity flow, whether it's paper, fabric, wood, clay, metal or various other materials, you can let your own imagination run wild or get inspiration from the numerous crafting instructions in countless books.

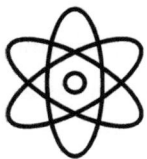

A few special suggestions:

Making homemade jewelry is not only a creative activity, but the results can also be used as gifts and bring a lot of joy. There is a huge range of beads (wood, glass) that can be connected with different types of string, and jewelry wire can also be used.

Homemade flowers made from paper, fabric and other materials (e.g. wire and varnish) not only help you to relax when making them, but are often loved as gifts.

The production of enamel jewelry and accessories is somewhat more complex, as is the production of small bowls and containers, also made of enamel. As a rule, this requires a steady hand and a somewhat elaborate kiln.

Self-made business cards, invitations and greeting cards can be a joy for the crafter and fun for the recipient. There are no limits to the imagination.

In the field of music, there are also no limits to what you can do. Countless instruments offer the opportunity to practice and be active. And anyone who enjoys singing, even if their voice is not enough to make them an opera star, should make use of this organ, because with the right breathing technique, singing is also very healthy in many respects.

Singing bowls are easy to use and are suitable for meditation and relaxation.

Homemade instruments, such as sound elements made of wood or other materials, and glasses filled with water are also ready for creative use and encourage creativity.

However, it is not only the creative use of sound and tone, but also the enjoyment of listening that can enrich the soul and promote relaxation, and there are many ways to make use of meditation music or any other musical performance.

Individually, there is also the possibility of addressing the rhythm, with music and gymnastics, with music and dance, there are also no limits to the imagination.

Walking, jogging and all sporting activities also allow the body to be creative or even work out. Mental sports are also a good way to relax; you don't necessarily have to go to group sports, there are short videos on the internet that provide instructions and, last but not least, you can consciously connect with your own feelings while doing your own movements.

A small example: Want to let off steam? Dance to the appropriate music and

create your own wild Tarantella moves!
Rock 'n' roll or twist are perfect for
working out.

Do you want to relax harmoniously and
mildly? For quieter relaxation, put on a
soft blues, for example with a gentle
song by Louis Armstrong within earshot!

Feel the music, feel the rhythm! Just let
yourself swing along!

You will also find a rich repertoire of the
most diverse melodies and rhythms in
all classical music, which can satisfy all
your desires for a gentle or spirited
mood.

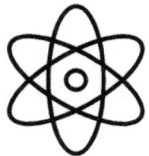

A few advantages and disadvantages of high sensitivity.

A highly sensitive person can tolerate less stress, as all impressions penetrate much deeper into their senses (deep-sensory).

He is often overwhelmed by this and has to de-stress. This usually has to be learned first. Because most highly sensitive people have not yet learned to find and draw their own boundaries, they constantly put themselves under pressure to perform and try to conform to the rest of humanity and orient themselves towards them and their performance.

This then leads to failure and disappointment, often setting off a large, negative cycle.

Highly sensitive people want to keep up with the others and set themselves far too high goals for success, even when they are still in a weakened state.

This constant stress then often leads to mental disorders, anxiety disorders, panic attacks, burnout and sometimes additional physical disorders such as headaches, migraines, tension, visual disturbances, dizziness, back pain, gastritis and stomach ulcers, etc., making it necessary to visit specialists and therapists.

In these and in all less serious cases, it is important for highly sensitive people to first get to know themselves and their own needs.

With very small goals, he has to try out what is good for him and how far he can go with his strength (nerves/body).

He should learn to pay close attention to the reactions in the psyche (feelings) and to see and recognize the reactions of the body.

It is important for everyone to find out how much stress they can tolerate. Since it is known that there is also healthy stress, it is important to test small stress situations in every form.

A number of medical methods have been developed for relaxation through conscious tension and relaxation. There are accompanying CDs for the muscle training methods. You learn to tense your muscles and relax them again. You start with the hands, which are tensed, work on the whole body and end with the feet, also with tension, then you follow this path backwards, starting with relaxation at the feet and ending with the hands. When you tense up, you create positive stress. Later, when you relax, you learn to use your muscles to relax the stress.

After a good workout, you can also do these relaxation exercises mentally (without visibly moving. A good exercise for on the go, also ideal in the waiting room) The CDs with instructions are offered everywhere, even by a health insurance company)

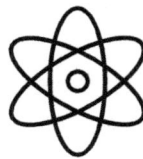

What is positive stress?

We feel it when we are happy about a task that we know we can accomplish. We can be happy and still be excited, aroused. We are tense, but this is not harmful.

Intensive, difficult work that we enjoy can put us under healthy stress.

Unhealthy stress often puts the psyche under pressure to perform, sometimes combined with negative expectations (of ourselves, of others).

Everything has to be done quickly and we are afraid of not being able to do our work, of not being able to do it well.

We want to do everything right and want to complete our workload satisfactorily for everyone, even if we are put under stress. We want to prove it to ourselves and to others. We set our own standards high or allow ourselves to be forced to meet the demands of others, even if they are too stressful, too high.

We want to be fast and good and prove to those around us that we are strong. We stress ourselves out when we demand too much of ourselves.

In the workplace, pressure is also caused by strangers who put us under stress. Highly sensitive people often allow themselves to be stressed in order to avoid getting into even greater difficulties. They want to do their job satisfactorily, be good, keep their job, and many people allow themselves to be stressed to achieve this.

Not all stress is avoidable, which is unhealthy for everyone, but sensitive people in particular need to make sure they have enough balance.

There are different situations and different types of stress and pressure that weigh us down. If we are forced to do something too quickly, this stress is obvious.

There is also emotional stress, which is less easy to recognize. It is offered to us in the interpersonal sphere and we can learn not to get involved in it.

We can avoid letting it stress us out by becoming strong and self-confident.

A small example:

Tina and Maria are friends. Tina has another friend: Lena.

Maria feels left out when Tina does something alone with Lena, she is jealous.

Tina loves crime movies, Maria loves romantic movies.

Tina invites Maria to the movies to watch a crime movie.

Maria doesn't like crime movies, she doesn't feel good watching them. But she accepts Tina's invitation to do Maria a favor, to please her friend and not lose Maria to Lena.

Tina acts against her own feelings, just to please her girlfriend, she puts herself under pressure to do something that is not good for her.

This example can be translated into all situations and groups of people, for example:

Child and parent

Friends among each other

Couples with each other

Employers and employees

This example is about pleasing someone else and putting yourself under stress in the process.

Of course, life in the community is not possible without compromises, but highly sensitive people in particular should check how much pressure they put themselves under when they give in to a fellow human being/partner more than is good for them and neglect themselves and their own needs.

Emotional pressure and psychological pressure are often underestimated because the negative effects are not always felt immediately, as the unpleasant after-effects (headaches, dizziness, pressure on margins, etc.) are sometimes only felt once the tension has subsided.

You are forced to look back at the situations that caused you stress and harm. This is not always easy, as you don't always recognize the pressure immediately and sometimes don't see through the situation straight away.

In fact, many highly sensitive people also "get used" to this constant stress because they want to "function" and don't take stress so seriously.

The stressful situation is perceived as "normal" and the highly sensitive person feels bad and inferior because they always feel like a disruptive factor or a failure who cannot fit in and adapt.

To do this, he should keep reminding himself that high sensitivity is not an illness, but a special predisposition that he and others should take into consideration. He should realize that this special disposition is intended by nature.

As a positive balance, he can always remind himself that this predisposition has given him great talents such as empathy and sensitivity, which can enrich his life.

In the meantime, many self-help groups and smaller associations have been set up to help this group of people and improve the lives of highly sensitive people.

Many professions have also begun to discuss how and where highly sensitive people can be deployed in a targeted manner so that this group of people can pursue the best goals with their predisposition.

I am referring to a documentary on the TV channel 3Sat, in which, among others, a contributor from the police spoke about suitable options and reported how it would be good to integrate more sensitive people into police work in a meaningful way in the future, as there are various professions in which empathy and good intuition are required. Other professions are also starting to think about employing empathic people in special positions.

And that brings us to the benefits that highly sensitive people can enjoy.

In many social professions, empathy is in great demand, a feeling, a good gut instinct, intuitive behavior can lead to success in many professions (for example in all medical professions such as doctors, nurses and geriatric nurses, therapists of all kinds, etc.).

And yet what is fundamentally important for all highly sensitive people also applies here: your own mental, nervous and physical health should not be overestimated.

The type and number of working hours must be adjusted individually.

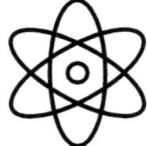

The greatest advantage that a highly sensitive person has is the following:

With his mindfulness, he is often already used to paying attention to his bodily functions, and even if he has not yet discovered this mindfulness for his body, he has the opportunity to **connect mentally with his body**.

The first trial experiences in the area of "body control" can be discovered during breathing exercises. You measure your blood pressure and pulse and note down the blood pressure and pulse data.

Then start a small series of 6 deep breaths: take a deep breath in with your mouth closed, then - without pausing - breathe out deeply and for a long time with your mouth open until you feel the sensation of breathing out in your stomach and upper abdomen.

If you then measure your blood pressure and pulse again, your pulse has calmed down and your blood pressure has dropped a little. This shows that you yourself have the power to influence your body (also "mechanically").

We try this in a similar way when walking fast: First, we measure and record our blood pressure and pulse rate. After walking fast or climbing stairs, our blood pressure is higher; if we measure it again shortly afterwards, our blood pressure is lower than before our activity.

A highly sensitive person also has the ability to mentally "govern" their body.

Once we have perfectly mastered the body's relaxation exercises (there are many CDs available, including one from a well-known health insurance company), we no longer have to perform them with movements, but can mentally instruct our body to perform these tension and relaxation exercises.

Relaxation journeys and other mental training also show us how closely we are connected to our body and how quickly and well it reacts to us.

With high sensitivity, we feel the connection between body, psyche and soul more quickly and intensively, can communicate with our body more easily and quickly, train it, "govern" it.

As a highly sensitive person, you can quickly find a better connection to your body and initiate a good self-healing process for minor disorders.

When psyche, soul and body are in harmony, the body can recover better and faster from stress.

Example: Headaches

A few years ago, I suffered from severe migraines, which were very troublesome for me.

After a doctor prescribed me a migraine medication, which I always carried in my pocket, the attacks reduced and soon disappeared. The fear of migraine attacks alone had made me more susceptible to them.

In the time that followed, I got headaches from time to time. As I have an aversion to medication and only take them in extreme emergencies, I started doing relaxation exercises when the headaches started. When I felt how well

I responded to relaxation exercises, the headaches also subsided.

It is important to realize how closely the psyche, soul and body are connected. If they are in a harmonious unity, small problems can be solved more quickly through self-healing.

Warning:

Of course, this does not mean that you should refrain from going to the doctor. Always have yourself examined by a specialist and clarify what health problems are present. Behavioral therapists and psychotherapists should also always be consulted before you are allowed to support your disorders with self-treatment.

Little by little, you will enjoy seeing how helpful it can be to communicate with your body, pay attention to its warning signs and help it with your own strength.

It is not only good for self-healing to feel deeply, to sense deeply, to think deeply, but also to be able to perceive and enjoy life more intensely.

It is a special gift to be able to draw strength from nature.

It starts with your eyes. When you look up at the sky and watch the drifting clouds, you can mentally open yourself to this image. You can feel the vastness of the sky, take it in and experience a liberating feeling. If you also breathe in and out deeply, you can intensify the effect.

Eyes are not called the "windows of the soul" for nothing, with them you can receive and absorb insights and views. When you look at nature, you can also focus on different colors that convey different feelings to you.

It is generally said that the color green is generally good for the eyes and can help you relax. Walks in nature are also very nourishing for the soul. Try it out for yourself! Try out how the different colors make you feel!

If you see a colorful picture in nature and have a little practice, you can also "drink" the colors. A color that you like or a colourful image that makes a positive impression on you can be absorbed by your soul and you can internalize it. Choose a few colors and images every day that you look at intensely with joy and let into your soul!

When you are close to the water, it can give you all kinds of different feelings. A clear, bright body of water triggers different feelings in you than a dark, shimmering, stagnant lake. A large, wide river, whose steady waves carry a relaxing melody, triggers different feelings in you than a rushing torrent or a waterfall glistening in the sun. Choose the sights that are good for you, that you like.

Not everyone has a river or a waterfall nearby, but you can find short documentary films all over the internet for free to give you a positive boost or relax you.

Check yourself, your feelings, note your preferences and consciously choose what is good for you!

The nose is also a very special organ. Many highly sensitive people have a good nose, which also makes them sensitive to unpleasant odors. But if you live in the middle of a city, for example, you don't often have the opportunity to help yourself to the pleasant scents of nature. Nowadays, however, it is also possible to buy the scents of flowers and plant extracts, where you can also try out what you like.

Some experts speak of fragrance therapies, so it is actually good for body and soul to enjoy your own favorite scents for a short time and let your soul participate in them.

Some people have a good memory for scents and like to remember good times from their past. Reviving these smells is also a good idea. Pursuing it can have a positive effect on your health.

All our senses are connected to our soul and can bring it good things.

On previous pages, I have already spoken about the music that can do our soul good. So we can delight and pamper our ears with the sounds, melodies or noises that do us good.

Not everyone has the opportunity to have melodious church bells or the singing nightingale nearby. I also refer to audios, CDs, films and documentaries.

Being woken up by an alarm clock with birdsong or a pleasant melody is healthier than being woken up by a buzzing noise.

The hearing of a highly sensitive person is more sensitive, unpleasant noises disturb them more, but the soul also has a very intense pleasure that positive sounds can give them. Choose your favorite melodies and find out which sounds make you happy!

You will certainly know how best to indulge your sense of taste and your taste buds. Consciously enjoy the food and drinks that you like! If at all possible, enjoy them in a pleasant atmosphere and harmonious surroundings. Whether alone or with nice people, try to turn every good meal into a celebration! That way, not only your body but also your soul will enjoy it.

You are probably also familiar with the possibility of enjoying several senses at once. For example, a picnic in the countryside, where you can enjoy something tasty, look at nature and listen to the birdsong.

Your favorite movie at the cinema or at home on the couch or in bed can become a small celebration with a few treats.

A visit to the theater, enhanced by a glass of sparkling wine during the interval or a good meal in your favorite restaurant, is also a multiple pleasure for the senses.

However, it is important that you find out for yourself what is good for you, what does you good, what indulges your senses. This can also mean a day of boredom or a day of lazing in bed.

In all of this, it is very important that you take yourself very seriously. Many people, especially highly sensitive people, focus their lives on others, on others.

They want to do everything right, they want to please others, they want people to have a good opinion of them. This applies not only to the professional sphere, but also to the private sphere. A person wants to communicate with others and be respected by them. Highly sensitive people often lack self-confidence, which means that they are increasingly dependent on the opinions and praise of others.

However, as you can't please everyone and can be both manipulated and exploited with this desire, highly sensitive people often find themselves in danger of immediately going overboard in many respects in order to find the right echo, the right resonance for themselves.

They are willing to work harder for their employer, to work a lot of overtime, possibly even unpaid overtime, to fill in for others and often to do a "favor" for someone else. By doing a "favor", you do what the other person likes and you find the opportunity to please yourself. Many people use this behavior to boost their self-confidence, whereas healthy self-confidence means being at peace with yourself without having to prove anything to others.

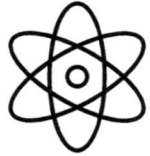

Different types where high sensitivity is a particular issue:

The order fanatics

Anyone who wants to do everything 100% all the time and who has problems letting things go once in a while has a desire for a perfect world, which, as everyone knows, does not exist.

Many highly sensitive person suffers from the fact that it is impossible to keep things tidy in the long term. I have met people who are upset that new dust is created every minute. These people have told me that they want to spend the whole day chasing after dust, literally fighting it.

Ideally, everything should always be harmonious, tidy and clean. But life is movement, ups and downs, everything is in constant upheaval.

Matter on earth is constantly in a state of transformation and one of these phases/states is dust. It is therefore just as much a part of life on earth as all solid, large material things.

As we all know, humans are also constantly changing, renewing themselves and their cells, skin flakes fall off and also turn to dust.

This renewal is a sign of vitality, also of ever-recurring life. It is important to be aware of this constant change and to accept it.

The hypersensitive person often desires the snapshot, the still image, which is a mirage, an illusion and has nothing to do with life. However, this desire arises from a longing for order, cleanliness, perfection and harmony.

This highly sensitive type of person suffers greatly from the imperfections of human life.

How can he help himself?

Just as every person can create a little paradise for themselves, this highly sensitive type can also create a field of activity and/or a little oasis in which they can build up this order on a small scale (in their home, their personal corner).

If he is able to, he should look for a job (or hobbies) where he can organize or tidy something. It starts with physical activities such as cleaning and extends to the areas of mental organizing, cataloguing and sorting. Anywhere in life where you can organize something, this type of person will be welcome because of their thoroughness and dedication. In the right place, he may discover that his extreme love of order is of great benefit and indispensable.

So as long as this person has his field of activity, he can also allow the forces to flow within him.

Nevertheless, it is important that he visits a counseling center if he suffers from his predisposition.

For example, there are extreme, pathological symptoms of a development that require treatment, such as a compulsion to wash.

A therapist can clarify to what extent such a predisposition is within the normal range and whether and to what extent there is a disorder that needs to be treated.

As a rule, oversensitive people who chase after constant order need a lot of security in their everyday lives. Sometimes this is due to childhood experiences, a lack of order, a lack of security or an imposing role model of sterile order.

In this case, it helps to review your existential and emotional security in your current life and work on it if necessary.

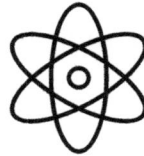

The anxious type

The anxious type worries a lot. As a rule, he thinks a lot and always wants to have everything under control. He thinks and plans and often calculates not only the risks of his own actions, but also the risks of the circumstances and the risks of the actions of those around him. He is sometimes afraid of spontaneous decisions and would rather have time to think things through carefully.

Planning means a lot to this person. It is important for him to know as much as possible about what is coming up as early as possible so that he can prepare thoroughly for everything. He wants to avoid risks as much as possible and therefore has an aversion to anything too spontaneous.

He loves clear agreements and rules and all things for which he can prepare himself thoroughly. Anything new is initially suspicious to him, and he is often afraid of new things. Stability is a very important issue, because he trusts things he knows. He even copes well with negative situations if he has practiced and knows how to deal with them.

Unfamiliar things and situations, on the other hand, frighten him because he believes he is not sufficiently prepared.

His main goal is not to make any mistakes, to do everything right, and therefore he prefers to do everything calmly, with great care and consideration.

Hecticness makes him nervous, hecticness gives him stress, and stress can then degenerate and lead to all kinds of anxieties.

As a rule, there were also people in his childhood who did not offer him any security or made him feel afraid.

At times, he was also forced to care for other people and bear responsibility for others. He was often overwhelmed by this and had to neglect himself in return.

This type also tends to view their own health with anxiety and alienation.

Even small things, minor irregularities in the physical sphere, make him fear that he is carrying major and serious illnesses within him, to which he is powerless. As a rule, he does not feel capable of having a good relationship with his body, but rather that his body could, practically like an overpowering force, bring him surprising, serious illnesses.

Every reaction of the body is viewed with suspicion, observed, it is seen as a powerful conqueror or even an enemy. In this latter situation, the hypersensitive person is in a state that should be guided into regular channels by a specialist therapist.

In a state of illness we find phobias, anxiety, panic attacks, bulimia, etc.

*

In the "normal state" of high sensitivity, the anxious person uses their own confrontation therapy. He confronts the things he is afraid of, he deals with these issues and the background, whereby therapists can also provide useful help.

The word **anxiety is** related to the word **tightness**. It is not uncommon for anxious people to feel tightness in the chest, respiratory tract, stomach or even a constricting "lump in the throat".

Tightness, distress, pressure, constriction, bottlenecks that are caused by circumstances or that highly sensitive people cause themselves, for example through the pressure of a disproportionately strict inner conscience, lead highly sensitive people into enormous stress.

If the external circumstances cannot be remedied or reduced, it is necessary to become aware of this situation and take countermeasures. To do this, the stressed person should find and implement their own personal anti-stress program (see above Sport and hobbies to combat stress).

Ultimately, a gentle form of confrontation therapy, a gentle familiarization with the anxiety issue and the associated increase in self-esteem helps to overcome any anxiety. **The aim is to become certain that there is a solution to most problems that arise in the future.** You may not find them on your own, but in any case there are helpful people and institutions everywhere who can assist you in overcoming problems. As long as the anxiety has not yet become pathological, a stable faith will also help you to develop a certain serene philosophy of life.

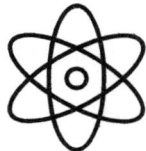

The you-man

There are people with strong empathy who neither want to be alone nor can be alone.

They have the ability to put themselves in other people's shoes in such a way that they can sense what is good for others and what is not. They have the ability to mirror other people or even slip into the role of the other person.

This ability is also found, for example, in actors, in some therapists or in people with similar activities where an understanding of the "you" is required.

It is an advantage for the detective inspector to be able to understand the perpetrator's ideas and intentions.

It is an advantage for a defense lawyer to be able to put himself in the defendant's shoes as well as possible.

It is an advantage for an actor to be able to put themselves completely in the shoes of another person. This ability can also be useful in the community because it can improve the social fabric. People who understand each other better can deal with each other and live better together.

You can understand each other "blindly" and many then speak of a common "wavelength". In private life, this strong empathy can ensure a peaceful life and good coexistence.

However, for the sympathetic person who always feels drawn to the "you", it can become a disadvantage if he or she comes into contact with very strongly ego-oriented people and becomes dependent. As long as the "I-man" does not take advantage of this situation, remains fair and does not overtax the "you-man", this symbiosis may work, which has also often proved successful in the animal and plant kingdoms.

However, in the plant and animal kingdoms, both generally benefit equally from this constellation.

However, the you-man wants to give a lot and takes little. The I-man wants to take a lot and often gives less.

This constellation also harbors a great danger.

This can quickly lead to an unhealthy symbiosis, as it is in the nature of many ego people to always seek improvements for themselves. What the you-man sends out or achieves with love and empathy is taken for granted by the ego-man, who becomes accustomed to the pleasant situation and seeks further advantages. A you-man always runs the risk of being taken advantage of when he gets involved with an ego-man. This can happen gradually, develop slowly, but can also develop suddenly in certain new situations. The ego-person doesn't even have to be aware that they are taking advantage of the you-person. As a rule, an ego-man has the urge to take the quickest and easiest way forward and to use his strong will and great energy to make it happen. Mindful of his advantages, the ego-man has no excessive thoughts for the people along the way.

This constructed constellation is now a blatant example in "black and white", the cases that occur are usually in all shades of gray, as most people are mixed types.

It is important that the you-man constantly reviews his situation and finds out for himself whether he likes his "role", whether he enjoys reading all the wishes from the eyes of the I-man and fulfilling them.

The ego-man, on the other hand, thinks less about motives, let alone about an imbalance of give and take. For him, the situation is perfect, why should he worry?

Consequently, the you-man must learn to take very good care of himself and pay attention to his strengths and the balance in the partnership.

It is a well-known fact that opposites attract in partnerships. There are various reasons for this, including the fact that nature has had something to do with the history of reproduction. A person with diverse qualities and dispositions is more capable of surviving well. This attraction of opposites is interesting and sometimes positively exciting in a partnership. And since a person radiates a lot of their nature, which can be intuitively grasped by the other person, it only takes a few seconds to determine how a future partnership can be lived.

Here, the empathic you-man radiates his kindness, with which he wants to engage with the I-man, and the I-man immediately recognizes the opportunity of a pleasant togetherness that supports him in his progress.

This symbiosis can work if the you-man does not give up on himself, does not develop a helper syndrome and the ego-man holds back with his demands and shows consideration for the you-man, helping him in his own way.

Under certain circumstances, this symbiosis can result in a good team in which everyone plays their part. This could be the case in the partnerships of earlier centuries, when the partners had their own role and had to live it. The woman had to take care of the children and manage the household, while the man had to protect the family and provide for its existence. Here, everyone could concentrate on their role and live it out according to their dispositions.

A lot has changed in our time since then, but unfortunately not everything that is important has grown with it, not all the necessary changes have been made, and the division of responsibilities between the partners has had to be reconsidered.

It is therefore important to check the symbiosis of a couple's relationship; if necessary, a counselor should be consulted to determine whether there is a healthy give and take in the relationship.

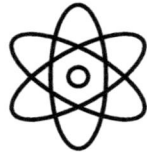

The fear biter

Different types of people have a very high level of sensitivity, which they prefer to hide because they cannot deal with it or are ashamed of it. Some of these types develop a defense strategy; they first check out their counterpart and test them. In doing so, they use their well-developed intuition to recognize the "opponent's" weak point. This strategy dates back to the early days of mankind, when competition still played a major role in survival.

Once the highly sensitive fear biter has recognized his opponent's weak point, he tries to tactically work on him, usually launching a communicative attack to test his opponent's strength.

This tactic is also frequently observed in the animal kingdom. For example, there are some insectivores that throw their victims, especially beetles, onto their backs first in order to expose their weak points.

As a rule, the fear biter has deep fears, hidden traumas that require careful treatment.

He tries to cover up his weak points by appearing strong and confident. As a rule, he attracts attention by trying to dominate other people so that they believe in his strength.

Sometimes he has all kinds of fears about life and needs a lot of security, especially in the existential and material sphere. In a relationship, he often does not believe that he is truly loved.

Some of these types of people feel that they are constantly unlucky and fear being left again and again.

This is why they fight with weapons that lead to difficult tests and even break-ups in a partnership:

In order to hide their own weaknesses, the partner is "belittled" by the anxiety biter. This often happens in communication, as the fear biter always finds a reason to complain about their partner or their actions. The more the partner allows themselves to be influenced, the fewer words the fear biter needs for their attempts at suppression. In a well-established, in this case unhealthy, symbiosis, a few reproachful looks from the fear biter are enough to threaten the partner and keep them down.

In this symbiosis, it is difficult to recognize that the fear-biter is an anxious, insecure and unconfident type of person. Exercising their power can nevertheless have an offending, sickening and destructive effect because this type of person always finds a way to weaken their counterpart.

As anxiety sufferers often act completely unconsciously, they cannot treat themselves but need specialist advice.

If left untreated, the fear biters later become frustrated people after a number of disappointments who, often unconsciously, maneuver themselves into a vicious circle of disappointment.

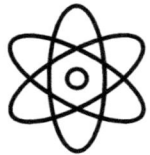

The restless, the hectic

The hectic and/or restless type feels inwardly driven to get everything done as quickly as possible. These types of people often worry that they won't get everything done in time, that they won't be able to complete everything, that they won't be able to finish something.

These people often try to do several things at the same time (multitasking) and start something in many different places. However, as they are often unable to continue working on every corner, they allow themselves to be pushed and disturbed by the unfinished work and projects.

They are often driven by an inner fear that sets them the goal of getting as much done as possible, as quickly as possible. Unfinished work often acts as pressure on this type of person; they often see their workload as a huge challenge that can only be met if they get as much done as quickly as possible.

This type of person usually needs a lot of movement and communication. They often have a talent for doing more than one thing at the same time, but there is always a risk of splitting up, getting bogged down, becoming completely nervous and becoming stressed.

The restless and hectic type, who is anxious when a large workload lies ahead of him, must learn to organize things one after the other and find a calmer rhythm in life. For him, the mantra "the journey is the reward" can be very helpful.

It is important for him to learn to value the importance of his work, his life force and his time. Focusing on the present is an advantage, so this type of person should see if they have any other fears about the future. Are they afraid of spontaneous changes? Are they afraid of strokes of fate (illness/death)?

Sometimes there are also fundamental existential fears behind this; this type of person wants to achieve as much as possible, usually to boost their self-confidence.

This type of person needs a lot of exercise, a lot of sport, to work out their inner turmoil. They often have difficulties with mental relaxation training at first, as they often don't find enough peace within themselves.

If at all possible, he can, for example, turn on calming music at home to accompany the activities that bring out his hecticness, or draw up a plan by setting himself the order in which he should do things.

This type of person should consciously realize that hectic and excessive speed often don't save much time. There are only a few seconds of time saved that are ultimately not used much.

In addition, hectic pace and excessive speed cause more accidents, and mistakes at work are often unavoidable during restlessness.

There are now even statistics on how little time you save by speeding. People often don't know what to do with the few minutes they save anyway. If you take a look at your daily routine at the end of the day, you can see how little the speed and time gained by rushing and restlessness can contribute to improving the quality of the day.

The restless type often wants to have everything under control at all times and therefore puts himself under additional pressure.

He doesn't like to hand over his work to others because he wants to prove that he can do everything on his own and preferably as quickly as possible.

This hectic type often only allows themselves free time when they have finished their workload and allows themselves few breaks, which means additional stress. As this type also quickly recognizes where something needs to be done, they always find something they need to start.

The bottom line is that they end up with far too little rest, far too few breaks and the additional pressure they put on themselves. Unhealthy stress is pre-programmed, so this type of person often suffers from anxiety disorders and stress-related nervous strain.

In this case, the restless and hectic type needs to see a therapist, and can also learn how to help themselves.

Every stress he faces must be countered by appropriate breaks and relaxation. Regular and good food intake is also very important for this type, as they usually don't even take enough time to eat in peace. He can take a very simple example from his daily routine.

In psychology, people are often compared to cars.

A car cannot run without gasoline. A person cannot exist without proper nutrition. He needs food not only for his body, but also for his soul, his psyche.

Even a car cannot be overstressed without damaging it. A human being is even more complicated and sensitive, and a highly sensitive person needs additional relief, stress-relieving hours and breaks.

This type of person must learn to pay particular attention to rest breaks in order to relax their overstimulated nerves.

Calmness is difficult for this type of person to learn; creative activity can speed up this process.

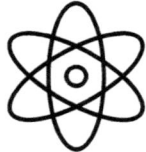

The hermit

This type of person generally feels most comfortable within their own four walls, where everything is familiar and they feel safe.

This highly sensitive person would prefer to do everything alone, preferably without the help of other people.

He often demands a great deal of himself and lives very modestly; he can also behave ascetically for long periods. He survives lean times and does not demand much of himself, neither from life nor from other people.

As a rule, he is hard-working, reliable, loyal and persevering.

He often develops anxiety when he has to be around lots of people, in the noisy hustle and bustle of a big market, an event, a supermarket, anywhere where there are large crowds of people.

This person often has very sensitive ears and cannot tolerate loud noises. With his special empathy, he usually feels an uncomfortable tension in crowds, which can also cause him to develop anxiety.

As a rule, he is friendly and helpful, but still likes to keep to himself so as not to become dependent.

He behaves cautiously and reservedly when he meets other people, sometimes he is suspicious, even fearful and is extremely slow to open up.

He does not take risks and loves the regular, familiar things in his life. Health problems often scare him as he fears losing his independence. He is rarely prepared to make spontaneous decisions, preferring to plan and keep an eye on his small, manageable world.

He often remains alone with his fears because he believes he has to deal with them alone. It is often the task of others to bring joy into the hermit's little world. Unfortunately, these people rarely go to therapy, so friends with whom they can communicate are very important.

This type of person is very resentful of their mistakes, has a strong to overly strong conscience and sometimes puts themselves under pressure to perform, not to please, but to please themselves.

This type of person should learn to see himself as a valuable creature, to feel that he can also have wishes that can be fulfilled.

Again, these characteristics can also be found in mixed types.

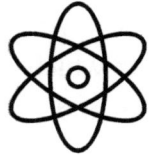

The panic attacks

In the course of my long life, I have met many people who have suffered from panic attacks at various stages of their lives.

Various forms of stress (physical stress, emotional stress, drastic life experiences, trauma, etc.) cause highly sensitive people to suffer from panic attacks at times.

For this form of anxiety attacks, it is important to seek the help of a therapist who can help with trained behavioral therapy measures.

These therapists also teach how you can help yourself at home, at work, in your free time, in everyday life, with which tips and tricks you can improve and change these times.

As I mentioned above, I also had this difficult time when I sought help from a therapist.

My experience with exercise, before and at the onset of such an attack, has proved its worth. Breathing therapy has helped me just as much as physical relaxation therapy, but I have also always tried to find my own ways and means of distracting myself in this unpleasant state.

The biggest problem for me was that I always felt like I was going to have a heart attack. I was afraid of fainting, passing out and losing consciousness. Above all, you could never predict how long such an attack would last.

In the beginning, I regularly went to a doctor during a seizure, who then found out from ECGs that there was nothing physically wrong with me. On the one hand, this was reassuring, but on the other hand, it made me feel very inferior and I sometimes had the feeling that I was going crazy.

It weighed heavily on me that I didn't have my body under control, that I feared fainting, that I felt **powerless.**

However, this began to ignite a rage in me that made me want to get my body under control again.

With the help of the behavioral therapist, who introduced me to all my fears and confronted me with them, I regained confidence in my strength and hoped for improvement.

When I realized that although these attacks were very exhausting, I was still able to survive them unscathed, I slowly and gradually lost my fear of fear.

I suspected that I could unconsciously push myself into these states of anxiety, but I realized that it must be possible to get myself out of this state again.

So I began to develop an intense feeling for my body, listening to all the signs in my body, especially my uneasy stomach feelings and my intense gut feeling.

I discovered that they must be important to me and gave me signals and that it was wise to listen to them.

At the slightest sign of an attack, I began to distract myself intensively, sometimes with quite banal tricks.

On the street, I counted cars with certain colors, people with special features or plants in the surrounding gardens. There was always something to distract me or count, so I avoided many attacks.

From this I concluded more and more that it may be possible to counter the attacks, to learn to govern and control one's own body.

As I gradually worked through the past traumas, I also allowed my soul/psyche to process the memories, but aimed to bring the recurring attacks to an end.

For this work you need time, patience and the help of the therapists (only the 3rd therapist worked out the final success with me).

I also remembered my migraines and that I could prevent them by taking a pill immediately after the first signs. I also remembered that they disappeared completely when I lost my fear of migraines.

So my most important goal with the panic attacks was also to lose the fear of them.

The more familiar I became with these conditions, and after I realized that they were demonstrably not causing any lasting damage to me, the calmer I became. The more I paid attention to the body signs and worked with my body, the less threatening these attacks seemed to me.

I now communicate very well with my body, pay attention to my sensitivity and try to unload the unhealthy stress with sufficient relaxation.

I am no longer angry with myself for this sensitivity, but try to be mindful of it and let it flow where it can have a positive effect.

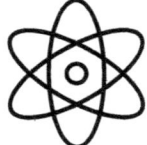

The consequences

Highly sensitive people are more at risk of stress-related disorders and stress-related illnesses. But don't we all know that people have their weak points? Doesn't one person often have to deal with a sore throat, another with neck tension or joint pain? With these complaints, people are used to taking care of themselves and protecting themselves.

How much more important must it be for us to protect our souls and keep our psyche healthy?

The word "psyche" comes from the Greek language and means "butterfly". When we think of a butterfly, the characteristics of a butterfly immediately spring to mind. First of all, we know that it is very light and can fly, sometimes it even dances while flying. It is very delicate, you don't like to touch it because it is very sensitive and you are afraid of hurting it.

When we think of our soul, we should also think of the delicacy of the butterfly and associate it in our minds with how vulnerable a soul is. Emphatic people who are highly sensitive are usually afraid of hurting other people and often treat them with care and caution. However, they often forget the vulnerability of their own soul and do not pay enough attention to the well-being of their psyche.

The generic term psyche also includes personality traits such as empathy and sensitivity.

This term also indicates whether a person is highly sensitive or less sensitive.

In the area of the psyche, we find that thinking and feeling are connected.

As a rule, the two "activities" are categorized under very opposing headings. Thinking is perceived as something very "factual" and concrete, whereas feeling is perceived as something sensual, heartfelt and undefined.

Here, highly sensitive people can gain a stronger connection to themselves and their psyche through a conscious connection.

Becoming aware-a combination of thinking and feeling:

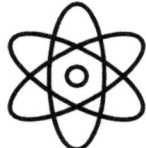

WE PRACTISE THE

REFLECTION:

I think about my feelings

I think about how I feel about life

I think about my feelings of love

I think about how my body feels

My senses send me feelings that I think about

I listen to my body language

My body sends me feelings that I worry about.

I can give my body instructions

(Example: when my head commands my hand to move, it moves)

(if I tell my body, even individual parts of my body, to relax, these body parts relax) see muscle relaxation training

I can give instructions to my feelings

(I offer you through the sensory impressions, for example through music, pleasant scents or special "moments". Take in this soul nourishment and feel a sense of well-being in your body).

With this profound reflection, profound sensing, the conscious connection in the totality of the psyche, I improve my body harmony, the harmony in the psyche.

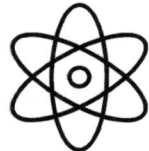

Unhealthy for highly sensitive people

are, as described above, the hectic pace, the unhealthy stress that we allow, but also the heavy use of the sensationalist press.

Of course it is quite normal to keep yourself informed about the situation in the world. It is good to be up to date with the most important world events, also to avoid being surprised by unpleasant things.

But I would like to issue a big warning for highly sensitive people to those who allow themselves to be informed by the sensationalist press and inundated with news all day long.

A constant stream of news can lead to nervous strain and anxiety, because the human mind cannot process such a flood of catastrophic news so quickly.

Many years ago, when people lived relatively isolated in their home towns, when there were no cars, radio or television, they were generally only informed about what was happening in their immediate surroundings.

People talked about it, discussed it and often processed it together.

In this day and age, the sensationalist press spreads catastrophes from all over the world, sometimes carrying them into our living rooms, and before we have recovered from the initial shock of the bad news, the next catastrophe appears.

Whether it's a train crash, an airplane disaster or events in a crisis area, all these terrible accidents are turned into day-long disaster documentaries in which viewers can participate at close quarters.

One would think that it would sensitize people if they could participate in the catastrophic conditions in crisis areas. They might sympathize and suffer and, in the best case, even be inclined to help on the ground.

However, with the amount of presentations worldwide, the flood of disaster reports unfortunately has the exact opposite effect. People become dulled and accustomed to such presentations, and highly sensitive people often carry the negative emotions around with them unprocessed.

Reports of wars and diseases, disasters and crises soon lead to additional fears. Where is it still safe? Who or what should I be afraid of? What can happen to me? How close can a war get to me? What can I do to protect myself?

Many highly sensitive people ask themselves these questions and are very worried.

Worried means that they are worried and afraid of everything that may come.

In fact, people have experienced all these terrible things over the millennia. My parents' generation experienced two world wars with all their atrocities and horrors.

We, all human beings, are aware that unexpected and terrible things can always happen here on earth, at any time.

But we should only worry about things that we can take care of!

The highly sensitive person must therefore check whether the issue they are concerned about is also within their area of concern. If you are a senior politician with authority, you may be able to influence an overarching event. If you are in a crisis area, you may also be able to influence events.

Most people, however, have little influence on world events (apart from demonstrations and similar opportunities to express their opinions).

If you make donations in kind or money for crisis areas or countries in need, you are in a position to help. So here again you have the opportunity to care for something, for someone.

Worrying about things that are not in our field of activity is not useful.

Unnecessary worries, worries that are useless and don't help anyone, are harmful and make highly sensitive people ill.

This means additional helplessness, which in turn creates a feeling of powerlessness.

We have already talked about feelings of powerlessness when we noted that many people with panic attacks are afraid of fainting.

So the average person feels powerless when they hear about war zones and crisis areas, which conveys fear.

Not everyone can drop everything to help in areas of need, so we need to be clear about where we stand and where we can help.

As a rule, we have the opportunity to care for something or someone in our place, in our everyday lives.

Sensitive people in particular like to take care of something or someone, as their empathy means they can immediately sense when someone needs something, and often even what they need.

It is not only in the family that there is the opportunity to care for other people, but also for friends, colleagues, fellow human beings in the immediate vicinity, animals and plants.

We can take care of something or someone close to us, and there are also situations in which we have to worry (existential hardship, illness, etc.).

Diffuse worries about something that might happen make us ill because we can't prepare ourselves for what might happen, we can't take precautions.

Worries that cannot influence an event convey helplessness and, in turn, anxiety.

That's why it's important to write down on a piece of paper what you're worried about, what you're afraid of.

Examine the individual points and determine whether you are worried about something that is beyond your control!

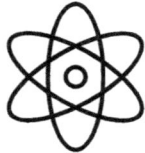

The feeling

We perceive with our senses. We receive sensory stimuli that evoke sensations in us.

Highly sensitive people absorb sensory stimuli intensively and can have great sensations that can evoke great feelings in them.

So it is no wonder that he can develop anxiety and greater fears when exposed to intense, negative impressions. We have already talked about the eyes, ears, nose and mouth, i.e. about seeing, hearing, smelling and tasting, and also about enjoyment, but we have not yet talked about the largest sensory organ, the skin.

People with high sensitivity often suffer from allergies, neurodermatitis or hypersensitive skin. The causes of these disorders can also very often be found in the burdened psyche and stressed nerves.

You can observe how quickly a highly sensitive person's skin reacts when exposed to stress.

A sensitive person's skin can react immediately to excitement and blisters, pustules or pimples can appear. Similar reactions also occur when you get angry or are exposed to other psychological stress.

Constant stress, constant anger, can promote chronic skin diseases.

Anyone seeking treatment from a dermatologist should also check whether and to what extent their psyche/soul is affected by stress.

The skin is also known as the most versatile organ that is useful and valuable to humans for various purposes. The skin is not only the body's protective covering that regulates body temperature, it also plays an important role in the immune system and metabolism.

There are receptors in the skin that allow us to perceive different temperatures and also pain.

In addition, the skin has the quality of a sense of touch and has a surface sensitivity with which we can absorb our sensory perception.

Highly sensitive people with their deep sensuality have the opportunity to develop a special sensuality that enables them to feel the pleasant "skin sensations" more intensely and positively.

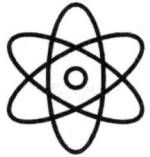

As you can easily imagine, it is extremely important for a highly sensitive baby to have a lot of skin contact, to be stroked and cuddled a lot.

It goes without saying that caregivers not only have the opportunity to feed, clean, apply cream, etc. They should also take plenty of time and rest to pamper the baby's skin.

Many adults of this type have experienced too little skin contact, too little stroking and too little cuddling in the first days and years of their lives, too little for their personal needs.

Everyone, especially highly sensitive people, needs good skin sensations, and there are various ways to pamper this sensory organ.

Let's think of a pleasantly warm shower, a bubble bath, an oil bath, a bubble bath! Let's think of moisturizing and oiling the skin, let's think of relaxing and pampering massages and, last but not least, of hugs between people!

Let us think of partnership and the touches in a loving embrace, in loving togetherness, in the experience of love.

It is well known that people who want to or have to live alone, unless they have other contact with people, often turn to a pet or other animal that they can get close to and touch.

We have long known how good it feels to pet a dog or cuddle a cat, and there are a number of therapies in which animals play a supporting role.

And what does a person who has neither a human nor an animal to cuddle do? As we know, they are advised to pamper themselves: with showers, pampering baths, creams and massages. According to the latest findings, adults should also reach for a cuddly toy that can be bought in toy shops, just like a baby or toddler. Various studies have shown that it is good for people to stroke something soft and feel the soothing touch. Soft cushions and blankets are also good for the skin and the body because the skin can pass on the soothing feelings to the soul as a kind of balm.

In nature, we can be caressed by a warm wind, a rough wind can free the soul from gloom and frustration.

Well creamed up, we can let the mild rays of sunshine gently warm and caress us.

On the warm beach, our skin looks forward to the gentle touch as we move in the soft sand.

A warm rain can caress our skin and refresh it at the same time.

When we touch large stones or hold smaller ones in our hands, we can experience various pleasant sensations.

Many people have already tried out how invigorating it can be to touch or even hug a tree.

We can try it out for ourselves, touch different materials and observe what sensations they evoke in us.

It is always amazing to discover how sensitively our senses react. If we test ourselves often, we can find out how "clairvoyant" we are.

Some people have an initial fear of contact with earth, mud and clay. Sometimes these fears can be traced back to childhood experiences. We develop our feelings of disgust and aversion at an early age, which are usually instilled in us by our parents. Here we should be courageous and slowly gather our own experiences.

You often see people playing with their jewelry in stressful situations or during

133

concentrated conversations: with a ring, a bracelet or their necklaces.

These touches can also have a positive supportive effect because they make our skin feel good.

It is important to test what is good for us and what is not. The more we get to know ourselves, the better we can deal with ourselves.

We can learn to focus more on the things that are good for us. If we know what is good for our skin, we can learn to pamper it. We can then pamper ourselves better after unhealthy stress and de-stress more quickly.

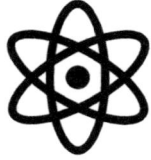

The creativity

We also find creativity in poets and various authors.

The privy councillor and lawyer

Johann Wolfgang von Goethe wrote:

Oh, that there are so many senses!

They bring confusion into happiness.

When I see you, I wish I was deaf,

when I hear you, blind.

Here, the famous poet mocks himself. Among other things, we know him as a very practical, very no-nonsense person who achieved a great deal.

He is also one of the highly sensitive people whose senses were particularly pronounced. Anyone familiar with his works knows that he was also capable of intense feelings, and the broad spectrum of his emotions can be seen in all variations: for example in romantic poems, vivid descriptions of his travels or the world-weary hero in "Werther's Sorrows".

With this example, I want to show that sensitive people are not weak by nature, but that they often allow themselves to be pushed into this role by their environment, which is different from them.

I also want to use this example to point out that this sensitivity doesn't necessarily have to stop you from going your own way to success and getting through everything.

You can have and show your strong sides and still have a high degree of sensitivity. You can be highly sensitive in some areas and consciously use your sensitivity.

This example also shows one of the many ways to be creative. Have you ever tried writing poetry, writing something, expressing your feelings in words? You don't necessarily have to do this for the public, you can describe something for loved ones or friends, you can also write something down for yourself personally.

If you feel like it, you can create a diary, let go of your feelings and thoughts or even let them fly. Have you ever read one of those strange poems that only the poet himself understands? And whether it's a small notebook or a thick book, you can even have it printed for a few euros.

You can write down the moments of your thoughts and feelings and record them in this way. They can become valuable memories for you and you will have the opportunity to follow your development again later.

In one of the sections above, I have already suggested that you simply try out everything that comes to mind in order to access your hidden creativity. You can also make notes about this, because if you don't want to pursue some actions yourself because you feel that you don't enjoy them, your attempts can give other highly sensitive people good ideas.

You've probably heard of people making things out of waste and scrap. In fact, there is almost no material that cannot be made into something new.

A few suggestions for you:

Old scraps of fabric can be used to make dolls, Punch and Judy figures or patchwork quilts, for example, while wool can be used to make toy animals without much prior knowledge by making round pom-poms, which can be used to create almost any stuffed animal. You can find crafting instructions on the Internet, but your own ideas are always welcome.

You can make creations at almost no cost if you collect roots and pieces of wood and take inspiration from their shapes.

Stones can not only be painted, but also used to build figures or sculptures.

Let's get back to the garbage. Glass bottles are turned into vases, painted, glued on, and the good old candlesticks, the bottles dripped with wax, are also timeless.

Even crown caps, bottle corks, tin cans, pickle jars and other packaging can be used to make everyday objects or small works of art in the form of sculptures.

Just take a piece of material in your hand, look at it, feel it and let it speak to you!

Many people lack the courage to realize their own creative ideas. As soon as they have an image in their head, they wonder what other people might think of it. Don't ask yourself whether someone else could do something with it, whether someone else might laugh at you or not take you seriously with your idea!

Not everything has to be serious and usable for others, and certainly not perfect.

Just have fun and try out what you feel like doing, discover what your feelings and thoughts tell you!

Take an example from the colorful, creative world that is full of surprises. And remember that every great inventor once started out small, experimenting for themselves. Don't give up the first time if it doesn't work! Creativity needs to be awakened, it grows the more you try.

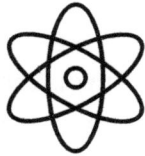

Quick help

If you are overstressed and anxious, you are in the best hands with doctors and professionally trained therapists. It is always reassuring if you can rule out serious illnesses.

But what do you do when you are standing at a checkout in the supermarket and you realize that you have a bad feeling. Of course, you can walk straight out of the store (without buying anything) or you can ask someone to let you in at the checkout. If you are brave and have experience with these reminders from your body, then you will know that it is telling you that you have taken on too much and it is time for a break. You don't have a glass of water to hand right now, but you can buy a bottle of water at the supermarket (or ask for a glass of water in other places).

This tried-and-tested remedy helps to release you from a tense situation. It is also well known that you should breathe in and out deeply in difficult situations. I recommend that you breathe in deeply several times with your mouth closed and then (without pausing) breathe out with your mouth open.

Do you want to prove to yourself that you have yourself and your body under control? Then, for example, remember a poem that you had to learn at school, hum a Christmas carol in your head and think of the words. But you are also sure to find some objects in your environment that can distract you when you are busy counting, as mentioned above.

Tell yourself that you can leave the store at any time or ask another person for help!

As soon as you feel better again, you can also thank your body for always communicating so well with you and giving you signs when you should take more care of yourself. Even if it sometimes sends you a warning when no danger is imminent.

You're also grateful for a storm warning outside so that you can protect yourself even if the weather isn't bad.

You can also learn to talk to your body. Praise it when it does something well, when you achieve something, even if it's not a huge achievement!

If your body sends you an unfounded warning, don't be angry with it, treat it lovingly and with a lot of understanding and patience!

Over time, you and your body can become a good team, you will trust each other, react sensitively to each other, and over time it will only warn you if there is a reason to do so.

What does that mean, the body warns?

In this day and age and in today's stressful situations, you have to learn to take particularly good care of yourself, your nerves, your psyche and your body.

A highly sensitive person requires more care. You can tolerate less stress and your nerves are more easily irritated. But the advantage is that you also notice more quickly when something is wrong. Your body notifies you more quickly and earlier if something is wrong to warn you. This is sometimes unnecessary, sometimes annoying and disruptive, but an early warning system also has its advantages. You can counter dangers sooner and faster. You shouldn't take the occasional false alarm too tragically! The more you do for your soul and your psyche, the more you strengthen your nerves, the more accurately your warning system will work.

There are people who sense climatic tensions, especially in changeable weather, thunderstorms, etc. Don't be afraid if you are a person who has unpleasant feelings such as weather sensitivity or negative feelings about certain situations or around different people! A sensitive person also perceives many different and diffuse moods in their environment.

Many sensitive people also have a strong connection to the phases of the moon. I keep reading studies claiming that the full moon, new moon and moon phases have no influence on people's well-being, but during my fifty years of work I have been able to disprove this in my studies. The number of inquiries from my clients is significantly higher at the full moon and much higher again at the new moon, with most of them telling me that they were much more restless at the new moon, which they often didn't even notice themselves. Sometimes they couldn't sleep at all during the new moon and were also plagued by restlessness during the day.

There are certainly many causes of restlessness and poor sleep, including late and poorly digested food, excitement in the evening, climatic conditions and, as we now know, the varying strengths of solar flares. Therefore, several components are always involved in poor sleep.

(See above for tips on how to sleep better)

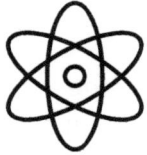

Dreams

Surely you know how important dreams are for you at night and that you can dream a lot during the different phases of sleep, even if you can only remember relatively few dreams when you are awake. Different types of dreams are known, lucid dreams, nightmares, true dreams; and everything that your psyche experiences during sleep is your dream life.

For meditation, I recommend, among other things, the oil painting by Pablo Picasso entitled "The Dream", which shows his young girlfriend as she sleeps.

It expresses a great deal of serene devotion with which you can confidently wish yourself into a restful sleep. It is generally said that there are methods of meditation that can both improve your sleep and help you remember your dreams better.

Dreams at night can say a lot about you, your situation and your mental health, and psychologists can advise you if you are looking for interpretations.

Are you also aware of how important your daydreams, your wishful thinking, can be for you?

The story of the little boy who starts out as a dishwasher and is always obsessed with the desire to become a millionaire is repeatedly mentioned as an example. This particular boy pursued his goal so intensively that one day he achieved it.

In order to realize your wishes, you should dream about them. Imagining something (in your mind) is also called visualizing.

With a fixed image (in your head) before your (inner) eyes, you can pursue a dream more concretely because you have a goal in mind.

When we set out on a trip with a specific destination, it sometimes happens that we tire in between and feel the need to interrupt or give up.

However, if we have a specific destination in mind that we are looking forward to, we can get through the tired phases well because we keep focusing on the destination.

If we have a clear picture of our dreams in our heads, it is easier for us to get through phases in which something stagnates or there are setbacks.

This applies not only to the realization of our private dreams, but also to the sensitive psychological constitution of a highly sensitive person.

In the various phases of his life, in which he suffers disturbances or phases of illness due to circumstances, it is particularly important to keep his goals for physical and mental health in mind so that he can pursue them more effectively.

However, it is important to set small goals in line with your sensitivity and not to be discouraged by stagnation and setbacks.

Set your goals! Write down your dreams and visualize them!

Wish for a harmonious interplay of body and soul!

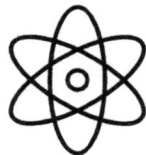

Self-love and love

Much has already been said and written about the topic of self-love, but I have to mention it again in the area of highly sensitive people because it is a particularly important topic for this type of person.

This group includes many people who identify themselves by their performance, who like themselves when they achieve something.

Equally common among this type of person are those who always want to be perfect and who resent even the smallest mistakes.

This group includes people who are very empathetic, like to help other people, are modest and often put their own wishes aside.

All these characteristics, which also suit modest people, often mean that a highly sensitive person first has to learn to love themselves

with flaws and weaknesses.

People of faith have it a little easier. They know that they are a creature of God who loves all people equally, just as they are, with all their faults and weaknesses. Being a beloved creature of God is something to be proud of. A mantra for all believers is the saying:

"If God is for us, who can be against us? (Romans 8 verse 31)

It expresses that we are loved and that we can feel worthy of being lovable.

Unfortunately, sensitive people have often not been told too often in their childhood by those around them that they are good just as they are, with faults and weaknesses. This unconditional love is not conveyed to every child. As a result, sensitive people often show a deficit in healthy self-confidence.

A trained therapist will be able to guide you on the right path, but you can also do a lot yourself.

I have placed the image of a white swan at the beginning of this chapter. Its symbolism contains the concepts of purity, light, beauty, majestic appearance, healthy self-confidence and love as the highest of feelings. The ugly young duckling in Hans Christian Andersen's fairy tale "The Ugly Duckling" also wants to be a swan.

Growing up among ducks, the little unsightly swan child feels more than just uncomfortable. He suffers from being different and his apparent ugliness as a result. The cute ducklings tease the outsider, so the young swan escapes. It is a long journey until, as an adult, he realizes in the reflection of a lake that he has not become a duckling at all, but a beautiful swan. Now he sees himself in the right light and accepts himself.

I relate this fairy tale to highly sensitive people who have not yet found their optimal path.

With all the wonderful potential that the sensitivity of this group of people contains, most of them see and feel themselves as disadvantaged outsiders, often even as weak people.

However, highly sensitive people have all the potential within them to become beautiful swans that respect and love themselves.

Realize that you are not only good the way you are, but that life has also wanted you to be this way with your rich "inner life"!

Being highly sensitive does mean being less able to tolerate some disturbing factors and experiencing all "negative" feelings more intensely (e.g. grief, loss, humiliation, depression), but you can also retain far more positive feelings for yourself as an essence in your soul. Joy and love can also enrich your life more intensely.

You are wanted the way you are. Be certain that there is a great secret, a mixture within you. Imagine the unknown day after your conception, when your genetic chain was formed, when it became clear what potential lay hidden in your personality!

If you are a believer, imagine the solemn day when your soul manifested itself in your body. A day that, despite well-developed science, can still not be determined today.

"This is how you were meant to be", say some poets who have already recognized how good it can be to accept yourself as you are.

Accepting yourself also means finding yourself good, and you can learn to love what you find good.

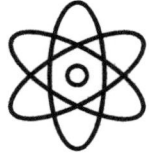

Love is a feeling that comes from the heart. Sometimes you also have to learn to love. Especially in nature and in interpersonal relationships, we can open our hearts and focus on our feelings.

"It warms my heart", people used to say a long time ago when talking about feelings of love. It is impossible to imagine many areas of love without a heart as a symbol. Let's listen to our "heart feelings"! Let's feel our "heart feelings"! Let our heart speak!

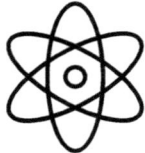

The word "self-confidence" means being aware of yourself, knowing yourself, knowing who you are. Self-confidence also means knowing what to expect from yourself. This allows a further step towards self-love.

Let's test ourselves, let's get to know each other! Let's find ways to use our sensitivity in a positive way. With the harmony we have gained, it is easier for us to find self-love.

Every person is an individual, even twins are not completely identical. Isn't it a fantastic feeling to be something that is unique?

Realize that you are not replaceable, because no one is like you!

When you move away from the duck yard like the "ugly duckling" and no longer feel like an outsider, take the path of your desires and dreams and goals so that the day comes when you can recognize yourself as a swan.

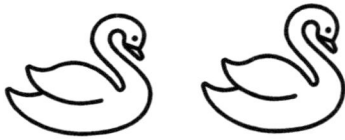

The highly sensitive person in a partnership

It is important for highly sensitive people to find a partner who appreciates the qualities and potential of high sensitivity, but who can also handle this sensitivity with care.

A highly sensitive partner usually has to find themselves first, discover their self-confidence and love themselves in order to find a partner who suits them.

Teamwork works best when tasks are divided up in such a way that everyone has their own areas for which they are

160

responsible and which they are able to accomplish.

As described above, the highly sensitive type tends to be very helpful to other people, even in partnership, but must be careful not to overdo it.

If he is with a non-sensitive partner, he should clearly state how much stress he can take and where his nervous and physical limits lie.

High sensitivity can be a problem, as the highly sensitive partner tends to take every statement, every word and especially every criticism from their less sensitive partner very seriously, which can put them under pressure and stress.

The highly sensitive partner often feels responsible for their partner's happiness and well-being, observes their reactions closely, takes many things personally and feels guilty when something is wrong.

In this case the highly sensitive type has to tell themselves that each person is responsible for their own happiness and that not everything can be shared, even in a partnership.

The development paths of the individual partners, which are necessary for each person, sometimes lead to a divergence. Partners who can communicate well with each other linguistically have a clear advantage. It is also useful to learn how to discuss or argue (also in couples therapy). But there are also moments when a hug helps.

As the senses of a highly sensitive person are extremely well developed, extremely empathic and receptive, the partners can, if they allow it, develop a great closeness to each other. There are no limits to positive touching, cuddling, massages, etc. All these touches are balm for the soul when two lovers connect sensually.

Because highly sensitive people are very empathic, they can often guess their partner's needs. This can have a positive effect. Unfortunately, however, they often assume that their partner has the same empathy and expect the less sensitive partner to show similar empathy and behavior. This usually unrealistic expectation then leads to disappointment. The sensitive partner assumes that they are less loved because their partner thinks and feels differently. This can lead to misunderstandings caused by false expectations. Each partner must be aware of what they can and should expect from their partner in terms of type and what not.

When you are given the gift of love, you cannot value it highly enough. Highly sensitive people also tend to immerse themselves in love and relationships, provided they have let go of their fears beforehand.

Sometimes they also idealize love or their love relationship, so the highly sensitive type should always look at the partnership realistically. When two people are together, compromises are always necessary, which can often only be found after difficult work. Everyday life awaits with constant problems and tests. Partnership requires constant attention and work, and it takes a lot of mindfulness to take love along this path unscathed.

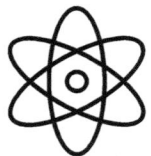

Moods

In order to treat yourself with love, it is important for highly sensitive people to know and observe their moods.

It is normal that a person who has slept well during the night is often stronger and more resilient in the morning. This makes them more optimistic and courageous.

In the evening, after work, and especially when it's dark, everything often looks a little different, sometimes less positive and you have less confidence in yourself.

The day offers many impressions, often so many that even a sensitive person cannot immediately sense what is good for them and what is not. As a result, they suddenly find themselves faced with a tangle of different feelings, feeling stressed and burdened without being able to clarify what has happened to them.

This is where the aforementioned helplessness and feelings of powerlessness set in again for many people, as they don't have the opportunity to take concrete action against anything.

Allow all feelings first! Accept them as a reaction to your environment, your experiences and then try to work out physically or seek mental and emotional relaxation! In moments like these, you can allow your soul to be disgruntled for a while. This means that it can't always be strong, courageous and optimistic, but is also allowed to "hang in there", to show that something wasn't right and that it needs a breather.

All feelings are allowed! It is good if you accept your feelings, anger, disappointment, annoyance and especially sadness.

Let all your feelings run their course, live them out as long as you don't deliberately harm other people with them!

For example, my pillow has always served me well as a boxing ball when I'm angry in times of grief and loss.

If you're in a bad mood, don't feel bad!

Life has enough problems and tasks that are difficult and require a lot of strength and work to overcome. There are also enough points of friction in interpersonal relationships that can cause anger.

Nerves are not fully resilient and a temperamental person sometimes reacts very quickly and strongly. If people freak out over every little thing, their nerves should be checked and treated. At the same time, you should get to the bottom of the causes of this temper tantrum (specialist advice) and possibly look for any traumas that may have triggered it. However, you can often find clues if you take a closer look at your childhood and parental home, which, together with a pronounced fiery temperament, can serve as an explanation.

It is also common to find people who initially accumulate a lot, too much, so that an explosive eruption of emotions occurs, comparable to a volcano.

In this case, the person concerned can learn to show their emotional reactions immediately to avoid getting into extreme situations. Behavioral therapists can help with good advice.

Many a plate has been broken during an outburst of anger by some people. In my large circle of friends and family, I repeatedly see people who, in small fits of anger, go after the paper waste they have accumulated. Shredding and tearing up cardboard and paper can help to let out the pent-up anger/rage of the day.

Joy should also be allowed, lived wholeheartedly. Everyone knows how healthy laughter is, especially when you laugh from the heart and laugh with tears.

From my childhood, I fondly remember a joke that we four children used to let my father tell over and over again because he could laugh the hardest and most heartily about it himself. Yes, then the tears of laughter would run down his cheeks.

Especially in this day and age, when people are under great emotional strain, it is important to find laughter again.

If you don't have the opportunity to be cheerful with other people, if you don't have the chance to observe the funny behavior of small children and animals, you can have fun with jokes that are accessible to everyone.

Laughing at yourself also needs to be learned. You can do it when you are "at peace" with yourself and have found your way.

It brings the necessary inner satisfaction if you accept yourself with your dispositions and talents, but always remain willing to work on yourself and learn.

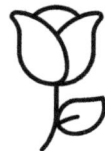

With the mantra:

I give what I can

(to the best of my knowledge and belief, even if I cannot always be 100% accurate)

you can look to the future with confidence and remain open to the bright moments.

Cultivate your positive feelings, hold on to them and remind yourself of them again and again! Learn to get rid of old ballast and mental burdens through relaxation exercises and washing rituals to make your life **easier.** Do you want to be happy with your sensitivity?

171

Strip away the old burdens, strip away your burdens, all negative feelings every day:

You can only fly with light luggage

If you are highly sensitive and have problems with it, first learn to deal with it in such a way that you can do yourself as little harm as possible! Know yourself well and take good care of yourself!

If you like, set yourself the goal of finding out for yourself why you have been given this special quality! High sensitivity can be a gift that enriches your life and can also bring joy to the lives of others.

This potential can bring a special meaning to your life and be a great help to other people.

Always avoid unhealthy stress and pay attention to your body's signals, through which your soul can speak!

If you want, set yourself the goal of using your potential to become a contented person who is profound and therefore able to lead a meaningful life!

Don't put yourself under pressure!

Live!

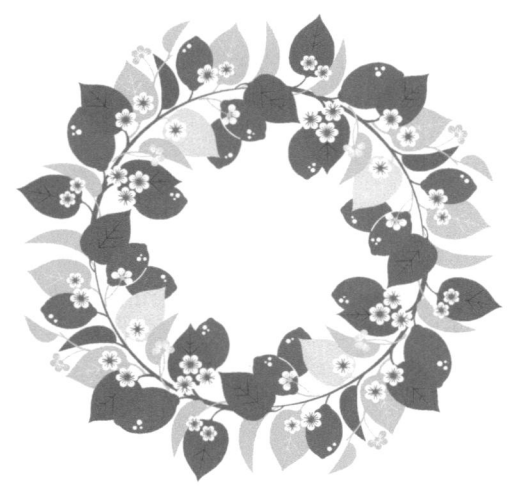

Here you will find space for your own notes: